MW01027296

Homemade Makeup and Cosmetics

Learn How to Make Your Own Natural Makeup and Cosmetics

by Lacy Stanton

Table of Contents

Introduction

With the advent of the organic, non-GMO, and other natural food movements, people have had a zeitgeist of realization about what we as a society are putting into and onto our bodies. More and more people are becoming conscious about the ingredients they're ingesting and making everyday use of. With this consciousness has also come interest in home remedies and homemade beauty products. In fact, did you know that most of everything that can be purchased can also be made at home with recognizable and more affordable ingredients?

When I first decided to make my own makeup and cosmetics, I was like a kid in a candy store, because, like most girls, I love beauty products. After years of spending more than my fair share of time (and money) in stores like Sephora and Ulta, I figured it was time to finally control what I was lathering onto my body just as I was already being careful about what food I put into my body.

Not only that, but if you have constant problems with things like breakouts, dry skin, or allergies, making your own cosmetics allows you to ensure that everything you use is something that is tailored to suit your specific needs. And if you're worried about time, remember all that time you used to spend in Sephora?

Now you're just using it for making makeup instead of shopping for it. Plus, once you figure out the colors and recipes you like, you can always double or triple the ingredients for a larger batch that can last you a relatively long time, taking into account, of course, the shorter shelf life of your natural ingredients sans preservatives.

All of the recipes listed here are so safe, you can even enlist your children to help. The experience will build up their creativity and also give you some quality family time. Who knows? You may like it so much that pretty soon, you'll find yourself starting your own cosmetics line.

In this book, I am going to cover recipes for skin prep (such as masks and lotions), as well as eye, lip, cheek, and bath products. And as a bonus, you'll also learn how to make your own deodorant!

Chapter 1: Facial Masks for Acne and Dry Skin

Facial masks are essential beauty care products, and people who use them feel that with their faces masked, it's like a day at the spa. There's also something really fun about running around with goop on your face for half an hour.

So, let's get started with an acne remedy facial mask. I just want to say first that there are a few ingredients that are super good for acne, and can be found in all kinds of concoctions online. They are, to name a few: honey, cinnamon, apple cider vinegar, milk, green tea, strawberries onion, and turmeric. What do all of these things have in common? They all have antiseptic and anti-inflammatory properties. The natural acids found in these foods will serve the same purpose as the salicylic acid and other ingredients found in store-bought acne cleansers, without the added harshness and irritation. In fact, things like lemons and strawberries contain salicylic acid naturally, in amounts not enough to be harsh to your skin. And the best part is, you probably already have most of the ingredients in your kitchen!

Acne Remedy

Did you know that you can make an acne remedy out of nothing but cinnamon powder and honey? Well you can!

All you need is:
- Some cinnamon (powder, not sticks)
- Honey (pure, raw honey, not the kind that's cut with corn syrup)
- A bowl
- A spoon
- Lemon juice (for later)

Raw honey is surprisingly easy to find. Just check your labels, and when in doubt, look in your supermarket's organic or health food section.

So, the mixture is one teaspoon of cinnamon to two of honey, give or take, dependent on how thick you want the mask to be. Mix it up, and apply the mixture to your dampened face for a quarter of an hour. Rinse it off when the time is up, and apply lemon juice as a toner. If you're afraid it'll be too much for your face, you can leave it off, but I would suggest trying it just to see how it affects you.

Vegan Acne Remedy

If you're vegan, and honey is off-limits, not to worry. Onions and oatmeal are all you need. The onion provides the acid, and the oatmeal acts as a drying, exfoliating agent to clean up clogged pores.

You need:
- One onion
- Half a cup of dry oatmeal
- Food processor

All you have to do is puree a good-sized onion with half a cup of oatmeal. The onion will provide the moisture to transform this into a facial mask. Apply it to your face for a quarter of an hour, then rinse and dry.

Next, let's move onto facial masks that will provide moisture for dry skin. Common ingredients used in moisture providing masks are also readily found in your kitchen. These include things like: honey, oatmeal, strawberries, cucumbers and avocado, and other fruits such as banana and grapes.

Dry Skin Remedy

My favorite dry skin remedy is so no-nonsense, so simple, it's a little bit crazy.

All you need is:
- Cucumbers
- Sour cream or plain yogurt

Use a food processor to create a pulp from the cucumbers, and combine it with some sour cream or yogurt. You want roughly one part cream to two parts cucumber. Combine and apply it. Let the mask sit for a quarter of an hour and rinse.

Vegan Dry Skin Remedy

All you need for this remedy is:
- One peeled and boiled carrot
- Half of an avocado
- About half a tablespoon of olive oil

Mash and combine the avocado and carrot, then add the oil. Leave on for a quarter of an hour and then rinse your face.

All of these remedies should be made whenever you want to use them, since they have all fresh ingredients. I would say that only the honey and cinnamon could be stored for later use. Even though these masks are all natural, I would not suggest using them every day. Keep a list of the everyday ingredients I've mentioned, and also try different combinations to find the most optimal combination for your skin. Just remember that for most, you will need one source of hydration, such as honey, milk, yogurt, et cetera, and one source of salicylic acid, such as fruit.

Chapter 2: Soft Smooth Lotion and Thick Cream

One of the most luxurious cosmetics, in my opinion, is lotion. The problem with store bought lotion, though, is that often they can get greasy, and no one's quite sure what all the ingredients are. If you make it yourself, then you know exactly what you are using on your skin. And you can make it with whatever smell or consistency you like. In this chapter are two lotion recipes. The first is a recipe for a soft, smooth lotion with the consistency of most store-bought ones, while the second kind is more of the hard kind, with exfoliating properties.

First, let's make the soft, smooth lotion.

Soft Lotion

You will need:
- 4 parts oil (any kind you would like; what does your skin need, and what scent would you like?)
- 15 parts liquid (again, consider what your skin needs. You can use any natural substance, such as water, tea, aloe vera, water, or any flower water)
- 1 part beeswax

- 4 parts coconut oil
- 4 parts cornstarch
- ½ a part of honey (if you like)
- An essential oil you love, or any combination of essential oils

Measure either by volume or optimally, by weight if you have a small scale. Melt all the ingredients together, save for the liquid and cornstarch, and stir periodically until the mixture is smooth. Warm up the liquid, and put it in a blender. Add the solid (wax) mixture, and blend until smooth. You'll know you're done blending when your lotion begins to become solid. You may also want to try putting the mixture in the freezer for a few minutes till it becomes firmer. Check every now and then if it has reached the consistency you want.

Hard Lotion *(Think face and hand cream)*

You will need:
- 3 parts liquid (same choices as above)
- 2 parts oil (same choices as above)
- 1 part beeswax
- 2 parts coconut oil

Blend them together in the same way as the first lotion recipe. As you can see, lotion is more work-intensive than facial masks or lip scrub, but it's still a lot easier than you might initially think.

Chapter 3: Lip Scrub and Lip Balm

Before we move into enhancing cosmetics such as lipstick and eyeshadow, I want to talk a little bit more about preparatory cosmetics. If you already love wearing lipsticks, you know how important it is to prep your lips. It's just as important as prepping your skin. That way, your lipstick goes on smoother and doesn't settle into dry grooves in your lips.

Lip Scrub

Lip scrub is one of the easiest and most satisfying cosmetics you can make from home. You need two to three ingredients. Just as with facial masks, you'll need a hydrating ingredient and an exfoliating ingredient. Commonly, the exfoliating ingredient is just plain old sugar. The hydrating ingredient can be petroleum jelly or any type of oil you like, such as coconut or olive oil. The third, and optional, ingredient is a few drops of your favorite essential oil, to give a delectable flavor and a nice scent.

Lip scrubs can be any combination of flavors and ingredients that you would like, and you can create all sorts of yummy combinations. The only thing that can limit you is your imagination.

Lip Balm

Lip balm is more complicated than lip scrub, because there's boiling and melting involved. For a basic recipe, all you need is coconut oil (or any other type of oil as you prefer), beeswax and if you want, Vitamin E. Vitamin E will help ease the chapping and can help to smoothen any scar tissue.

Here's your list of ingredients along with everything you need for measuring and mixing:

- Beeswax
- Vitamin E
- Coconut or other oil
- A container for your balm
- Measuring cup and spoons
- A grater
- A microwave (or you can do things the stovetop way)

You need two parts oil to one part beeswax, plus or minus a bit of either to achieve a preferred consistency. The final ratio of ingredients is up to you, depending on the batch size you want, but just make sure you use the base formula. Add a few drops of Vitamin E if desired. Before you can mix your ingredients, you'll probably need to grate your beeswax, and then combine it all. Melt the mixture in the microwave. Do it a bit at a time, taking it out of the microwave to stir it periodically. Next, you let it sit till it firms up and it's ready to use. Just as with lip scrub, you can add any essential oil or powder such as cocoa or cinnamon for flavor or color. If you don't want flavor, but you want color, try a tiny bit of red food dye. If you want colorless flavors, most essential oils will work well.

Chapter 4: Crayon Lipstick, Solid Lip Gloss, and Liquid Lip Gloss

Crayon Lipstick

Continuing on with the theme of lips, if you're an adventurous lipstick girl, this one's for you, although you may still want to prep your lips with a non-tinted scrub and balm. Not only can you make your own lipstick at home, you can make any color of lipstick at home by using crayons. This makes for some wild colors, a la Kat Von D or Melt brand. And the bigger the pack of crayons you get, the more conventional colors you'll have available to you as well. The reason crayons work just as well as a lipstick is because they are already a highly pigmented, wax-based, non-toxic substance. The amount of ingredients is based on a chapstick case or small tin. If you need more, just double or triple your amounts.

You will need:
- A mold, tin, or chapstick case to hold your final product
- A measuring cup (metal or heat-resistant plastic)
- Half of a crayon (or a quarter, if you want to combine colors)
- Half a teaspoon of jojoba oil, coconut oil, or other oil of your choice.

21

- A small bit of shea or cocoa butter

To combine these ingredients, you'll have to melt them, but I have a feeling using the microwave would just result in a huge mess, so, this is where your heat resistant mixing bowl comes in. Put all of the above ingredients in your mixing bowl and set aside. Bring a small, shallow, pan of water to a simmer, not quite a boil, and then place the bowl of ingredients in the water. Stir, using a wooden spoon or other implement to combine and make the mixture smooth. Pour the completed mixture up into your chosen container, and allow it to cool and set.

Your lipstick is done, and now you can be the proud owner of as many colors as Crayola can provide, and more, if you mix them up.

Solid Lip Gloss

Unfortunately, (or fortunately, depending on your preference) homemade lip gloss is much like homemade lip balm. It has the same base ingredients, like natural oils and beeswax, but there are some variations as to the source of pigment. Here is the recipe for you. You can always make both this and the balm recipe and see which one you end up liking better. If you're looking for a more traditional liquid lip gloss look, I'll include another recipe further down for that as well.

To make a solid lip gloss, you will need:
- Beeswax
- One or more types of oil, options including: almond oil, olive oil, or coconut oil—combine them or use them separately
- Any essential oil or a combination of essential oils
- Any color powdered blush and/or lipstick that you want as a tint
- A container for your gloss, and mixing bowls and spoons

Here's what you do: you take two tablespoons each of the beeswax, almond and coconut oil, and one tablespoon of olive oil. Add as many drops of the essential oils you want to the mixture. Add in about a quarter to half a teaspoon of the substance you'll be using as your tint. This depends on how vibrant you would like your gloss to be. Place some water in a mid-sized pan, and heat until it simmers, but not boils. Place the container with the beeswax and oils into the water, stirring until they melt evenly. Add your other oils at this point. Then add in your coloring at the very end, while the mixture is still hot, and stir until melted, as before. Pour the mixture into your container.

Liquid Lip Gloss

You will need:
- Petroleum jelly (e.g. Vaseline)
- Castor oil (this type of oil will make the gloss more shiny, though you can experiment with other oils as well)
- A loose powder eyeshadow or mica in the color of your choice

Put your colored powder in one bowl and in another combine your oil and petroleum jelly. Microwave or melt on the stove in a heat-resistant container, checking on the mixture periodically. Add the pigment to the liquid mixture, and stir.

You can find traditional liquid lip gloss containers at beauty supply stores, or you can store the lip gloss in little jars or other containers. If you have to do the latter, use a brush or cotton swab to apply.

Chapter 5: Basic Powder Eyeshadow and Cream Eyeshadow

I don't know about you, but aside from lipstick, eyeshadow is my favorite cosmetic product. It's so much fun to experiment and blend, and it can have so many looks, from metallic to matte, to a subtle shimmer, to super glittery. Just as with lipstick, you can make this from home, and who knows? You might love making eyeshadow even more than buying it. Just think of all the fun colors you can make.

Basic Powder Shadow

That's right, this is a recipe for good old pressed powder. Depending on what consistency you like, you could also use it for blush or eyeliner. Of course, that also depends on the colors you choose.

All you need are three components, which are:
- Powder base
- Mica pigment
- Powder binder (which can be bought as a spray)

You will also need:

- An herb grinder for the powder
- A container
- A mini-press to push the powder into the container (although a spoon works just fine as well).

Grind up and blend the mica with the powder base. And guess what? Here's the fun part where you mix colors of mica to create your own unique shades, and even add some glitter if you want it. If you like loose eyeshadow, you can stop there and store your powder in a jar. You might want to install a tiny sifter on top, though, so you don't spill it all when you open it to apply it.

However, if you do want a pressed powder, pour the mixture into another container and spray with the powder binder. Mix it until it reaches the desired color and consistency. Remove the eyeshadow from your mixing bowl and put it into its final container, where you will press it flat. Repeat until you've made all the color combinations you'd like.

Note: Arrowroot powder, which can be found in the health food section of your grocery store, is a good base powder to add to the mica. And, if you want a matte shadow as opposed to a pearlescent or shimmer shadow, use iron oxide instead of mica. You can also combine iron oxide and mica for an in-between, sort of "frosted" look that works well with metallic and cool colors. You may also want to consider adding a little bit of natural oil to make your powder adhere more easily to the skin.

Cream Eyeshadow

I so love cream eyeshadow not only because it provides a completely different texture from pressed, but because it can also be used as an eyeliner if applied with a tiny brush.

To make cream eyeshadow you will need:
- Beeswax, which you can buy in pastilles or otherwise
- Shea butter
- Jojoba oil
- Vegetable glycerin
- Vitamin E oil
- Mica or iron oxide pigment
- Measuring spoons and cups
- Container for your finished products

Measure out about the same amount of beeswax and shea butter, for example, about one teaspoon each. Or you can choose to multiply the recipe. Melt the wax and shea butter together, and add one part jojoba oil to five parts glycerin, and half a part of vitamin E. You may need to use a pipette (or dropper) for this part if you are making only a small batch. Measure out your pigment. Add less for a light, subtle color or more for a rich, vibrantly pigmented color. Stir all of the ingredients together and let sit a day in your eyeshadow pot before using.

Chapter 6: Natural Blush

There's no secret ingredient in making blush that's perfect for your skin. Even though I don't know too many people who wear blush (or rouge, as it is sometimes called) I figured it would be good to include it for those adventurous souls who would like to experiment with it. It works under the same principle as pressed eyeshadow, with a base, a pigment, and a binder if you want it, but of course with blush you would select a pigment that's more within the natural realm of shades. This is dependent on your skin tone, and can range from pale pinks and reds to oranges and deep browns. Because of this, you can use flower, plant, or spice based pigments over the mica or iron oxide component of eyeshadow. I would also suggest a natural pigment over these two aforementioned choices because in general, you want blush to be a matte pigment, or at the most a very light shimmer.

For your natural blush, you will need:
- Arrowroot powder (as before with the pressed eyeshadow, it will act as your base powder)
- Hibiscus powder
- Cocoa powder
- A container for storage

Note: Hibiscus powder and cocoa powder are just two suggestions among hundreds, if not thousands or naturally pigmented herbs and spices you could use to color your blush. In fact, in the course of my research for this book, I found a lovely site called Mountain Rose Herbs, which not only stocks the hibiscus powder, but also other herbs and spices such as anise star pod powder, which is a coppery orange in color, annatto seed, which is a deeper red, and beet root powder, which is more purple. What's also great is that if you're concerned about any allergic reactions, they've got you covered. With each ingredient is listed uses and precautions. With each of these pigments, you may have to experiment with how strong each one is and adjust the amounts of powder accordingly.

That said, back to the recipe. The base recipe calls for half a teaspoon of each ingredient, plus or minus more if you need it. So really, your amounts will depend on the size of the batch you'd like to make, as well as how pigmented you want it to be, as well as what combination of color you're using, if using more than one pigment. Remember that as you are combining your makeup, you should test it on your face or arm to make sure it's the shade you want. Also, less is more. You can always add more of a darker shade, but you can't take it away, so begin with the base amount and experiment from there. With your homemade blush, your cheeks will be all glowy and happy!

Chapter 7: Shampoos for Dry or Oily Hair

Now that I've covered quite a few cosmetics, I figured it'd be nice to mention some bath products, especially things like bath bombs and bath salts, because I know everyone loves to feel pampered. We all know that Lush is great, but they are kind of holding the monopoly on luscious bath products these days, and a trip to that store can result in a real bank account drain if you're as much of a fan as I am. Not only that, but things like homemade bath bombs also make such awesome gifts, a novel alternative to the standard gift baskets you find in supermarkets. Those baskets of commercial bath products often smell of chemical and are funky anyway, unless you're buying high end ones. But before we get to the cool stuff like bath salts and bombs, I want to mention that shampoo is also something that's wonderful to make at home.

If you have made shampoo at home before, (or purchased it from a health food store), you know that it doesn't get as lathery as regular store-bought, processed shampoos. That's because the majority of lather comes from added chemicals that react together to create the feel that we expect. Most of these shampoo recipes will not lather up a lot. In fact, smaller bubbles are far more effective than the larger bubbles of the regular foamy lather, so don't worry about your hair not being clean afterwards.

The good thing about making your own shampoo is that you can select the combination of ingredients to make something that will fit the needs of your hair exactly. In this section, I have chosen to include two recipes that work well for oily hair and two for dry hair.

Shampoo #1 for Oily Hair:

You will need:
- Baking soda
- Water

That's it, really. And you just need a tablespoon to a cup or two of water. Put it in an old shampoo bottle and shake it up. That's it, you're good to go. Not only is it good for excess oil buildup, but it helps to remove dandruff as well.

Shampoo #2 for Oily Hair:

You will need:
- Half a cup of Castille soap
- Teaspoon aloe vera gel (not juice)
- Two tablespoons of lemon juice

Shake it up and you're good to go.

Shampoo #1 for Dry Hair:

This one is insanely simple too:
- One cucumber
- One lemon

Peel them both, then blend them up until you've got a nice puree. It might take a while, especially with the lemon chunks. If you don't like the idea of having to pull bits of lemon out of your hair later (this can happen if it isn't blended well enough) then try using lemon juice instead. I would still recommend using one lemon's worth of juice.

Shampoo #2 for Dry Hair:

You will need:

- One cup liquid Castille soap
- Two tablespoons apple cider vinegar
- One tablespoon tea tree oil (tea tree oil can be very harsh, so if you've got sensitive skin, I might suggest using less, or diluting it with a bit of water until you know how it affects you)
- A quarter cup of water

Combine it all into an empty shampoo bottle or spray bottle if you would prefer, and apply to hair.

Chapter 8: Bath Salts and Bath Bombs

Bath Salts

Bath salts are so pampering and good for your skin as a natural exfoliant. Not only that, but it's crazy how easy they are to make, and they won't have any strange chemical smell to them, plus no unnatural dyes if you don't want them in there.

You need two ingredients:
- Bath salt
- Essential oil

Combine sixteen ounces of bath salt with fifteen or so drops of your choices of essential oil for a lovely scent. You can also experiment with the proportions for a stronger or lighter scent. I think it would also be super cute to add some dried flower petals, such as rose or lavender, and tie them up into little sachets as gifts. You can find bath salt by searching for it online, but an easy thing to remember is that you want a course ground sea salt or Epsom salt. Personally, my favorite is Himalayan pink salt, because it's so pretty and feminine.

Bath Bombs

You will need:
- Baking soda
- Corn starch
- Citric acid
- Essential oils of choice
- Food coloring if you want it

To prepare you will also need a spray bottle, bowl, and a cupcake pan, although it might be super fun to find some shaped molds, just for the whimsy.

Combine one and three-quarter cup of baking soda, one cup of citric acid, and two cups of cornstarch. This is your base mixture. If you want the food coloring, you add a couple drops to some water and add it to your mixture. You can use the spray bottle for this or just pour it in, whichever you prefer. Pour the water slowly, however. You don't want your mixture to fizz up before use. When it contains enough moisture to be tightly packed into the mold, do so, adding your essential oil of choice right before packing. As with every recipe here, you may need to experiment with food coloring and essential oil amounts before you achieve exactly what you're looking for. Let the bath bombs rest in the pans for a few hours before removing them. As with the bath salts, consider packaging them up in little sachets with complimentary flower petals or herbs.

Chapter 9: Under Arm Deodorant

Ah, deodorant. Of all the products I've talked about today, I feel that this is probably the most unexpected and potentially the most taboo. Every other product I've mentioned has something to do with pampering, not true necessity, and let's face it -- no one likes to think about sweat or body odor. You may be thinking that there are so many natural deodorants to be found these days, along with all the lovely scented normal varieties, so why bother making one yourself. You'd be right, but these natural store bought options can be way too expensive, more so than a stick of deodorant has any right to be. Not only that, but just as with every other products I've described, you have way more control over what goes into it. You know what that means: no more harmful chemicals going onto your armpits, and no more weird chemical stinky feeling.

To make homemade deodorant, all you need are four ingredients:
- Arrowroot powder (again)
- Coconut oil (yes, like the kind you cook with)
- Baking soda (to soak up that sweat aroma no one likes)
- Your choice of essential oil so you smell yummy

Start with one third cup of the coconut oil, and one third cup arrowroot powder, plus two tablespoons of baking soda. The amount and combination of essential oils is up to you, as usual. All you need otherwise is a small bowl and spoon, as well as something to store the finished product in.

Mix all the base ingredients (everything but the essential oil) together until you reach the desired consistency of deodorant. Then add in your essential oils. While I suppose you could make a bar out of this with some binder, it really isn't necessary. You can just apply it with your fingertips. If you think this is gross, and really would like a solid deodorant, just add in some beeswax and that should stiffen it right up. You'll also need to put it in a mold as it cools if you do this step.

And voila! A deodorant that is both safe and smells enchanting.

Conclusion

Now you know that making your own cosmetics is a lot easier than you initially thought. What makes things even better is you know every ingredient in the product you're using. As with all cosmetics, store-bought or otherwise, these should be made in small batches unless you plan to sell them or give them as gifts. You should replace your batch every two to three months. The amounts featured in this book should be enough for just that length of time.

Try experimenting with your oil and color combinations, and you might be pleasantly surprised at the results. Note down what worked and what didn't, so you'll know exactly what to do next time you make a new batch. If you give away some of your homemade beauty products as gifts to friends and relatives, ask them their favorites and why. This way, you'll know what products you have to make more of come next gift-giving time.

You'll definitely feel much better after excluding all those chemicals found in store-bought cosmetics. Making your own cosmetic products from the comfort of your own home is truly a win-win situation not only for your body but with the money you save, for your purse as well.

Finally, I'd like to thank you for purchasing this book! If you enjoyed it or found it helpful, I'd greatly appreciate it if you'd take a moment to leave a review on Amazon. Thank you!

Made in the USA
Middletown, DE
29 November 2016